Boy Or Girl? You Decide!

Practical Natural Safe Ways To Get Pregnant With

The Baby of Your Choice.

By
Nkiru Ojimadu

This is an

Ojimadu Books Publications.

Copyright © 2017 by Nkiru Ojimadu

All rights reserved. No part of this publication may be reproduced, distributed, or transmitted in any form or by any means, including photocopying, recording, or other electronic or mechanical methods, without the prior written permission of the publisher, except in the case of brief quotations embodied in critical reviews and certain other noncommercial uses permitted by copyright law. For permission requests, write to the publisher, addressed "Attention: Permissions Coordinator," at the address below.

Book.ojimadu@gmail.com

I dedicate this book to all women who have suffered different types of humiliations, from their husbands, society, families, in laws, etc, in search for a male child.

contents

What Others Say About This Book 7

Introduction 12

Chapter 1 23

How to get pregnant with a boy 23

    From Biology Class, We Know That... 24

    He Has To Wear Boxers 25

    Hot tubs and hot baths Are Your Enemy For Now. 26

    Take Cough Syrup 26

    A cup of coffee to the rescue! 26

    Consume more calories 27

    Know Your Ovulation Date 28

    Have sex as close to ovulation as possible. 31

    When does ovulation usually occur 32

    How do I know my ovulation date? 32

    How To Measure Your BBT 40

Ready to chart your BBT?..40

Don't like charting? Go for OPK (Ovulation Predictor Kit) 42

How To Use An Ovulation Kit. 43

Silva Test 43

In Summary - To Conceive a baby boy 45

Chapter 2 47

Sex Positions For Making A Baby Boy. Other Sexual Attitudes That Help You Make A Boy. 47

The Theory 47

Say Goodbye To Missionary Sex 49

Have An Orgasm 52

Chapter 3 53

Vaginal Alkalinity And Your Diet 53

Eat a Healthy Diet 54

Chapter 4 66

What to Avoid To Increase Sperm Count...66

Chapter 5 81

Supplements That Increase Sperm Count...81

In Conclusion 88

Chapter 6 89

16 Common Medications That Can Lower Your Sperm Count You Should Avoid. 89

Chapter 7 94

Summary Of How to Conceive A Boy 94

Ovulation And Timing: Do Not Miss This! 98

Remember: timing is the key! 99

Female Orgasm When Conceiving A Boy 100

The Father's Role 100

Douching 103

My Advice 104

Chapter 8 105

Methods For Having a Sweet Baby Girl 105

The Secret To Gender Selection. 106

How To Select The Right Time To Have Sex And Make Sure You Conceive A Girl. 106

The O +12 method (Ovulation plus 12 day) 107

Easy Sex Positions Which Highly Boost The Chances Of Having A Baby Girl. 107

Have a hot bath, both of you! 108

Eating for a baby Girl 108

Sex Positions That You Must Keep Away From, To Make a Baby Girl .. 110

Just Say "No" to the Big O 110

Cough Medicine Is Bad For Making Baby Girls 111

Woman Be In Charge On Bed During Baby Making Period 112

What Others Say About This Book

I love what I read. It was quite down-to-earth and so on point. Nkiru Ojimadu shared some truth that only the brave and contemporary thinkers would embrace. All in all, those who are meant to read it would grab it and run with it.

I can testify to some things which are both medically and factually correct like positioning, ovulation kid etc.

After waiting for 6 years between my first and second, I also got desperate and tried everything as a healthcare professional and some of the things you shared, I did. Solely though, it was divine intervention and Gods mercy. Naturally, according to the Doctors report, I wasn't even supposed to conceive let alone have kids because my ovulation cycle was not usual.

The book was Very easy to read and understand and it would challenge and blast traditional norms that says, "what will be, will be"

Or by the way, I was 32 when I had my first one and 38 with the 2nd, using a mixture of methods and the 3rd one (Joy) at 40+. She was the bonus and icing on the cake after waiting for long. If I had known all these things you wrote in greater depth like this, I probably would have ended up with a fourth child and had them earlier, so no one should ignore these tips if they are truly desperate.

Lydia Olorunniwo

Certified adult nurse trained in the U.K. With 25years nursing experience. Nursing Sister in Dermatology and Tissue Viability.

Advanced Nurse practitioner in general practice.

Orpington, Kent UK.

It works!!! I have two boys using methods and tips shared in this book. Now, I have 2 girls and 2 boys! You have no reason not to use the advice in this book. Most of my friends have used the tips in this book as well to get results. Recommended!

Uju Ojimadu Okpala, A Pharmacist, Fertility Coach.

As a medical practitioner in this field for more than 30 years, I recommend this book to all couples knowing that it will help families, especially in Africa, to prevent having lots of unnecessary pregnancies in search of a baby boy. Thanks, Nkiru for writing this book.

Dr. Osita Chukwuemeka Ekeh.

Medical Director

Chelsea Specialist Hospital and Maternity,

Nkpor, Anambra State,

Nigeria.

I used to have an idea of how a woman can produce her choice of baby, either a boy or a girl and I used to say it is not possible, but this book has really widened my knowledge on it and I have come to understand it is not as difficult as I have always thought it was. I therefore recommend the book to everyone and I believe we can help ourselves once we are informed.

Kolawole Oluwaranti

A medical technologist

I recommend this book to all couples in search of a child of their desired sex and also to all intending couples.

Folasade Evelyn

Registered Nurse.

If every couple had this book before their baby making, they would have done a lot of things differently. If you really want to be sure which baby to have, get this book. I have recommended it to everyone that I know need it.

Thelma Ibeh

A registered nurse,

CEO & Founder GlitznGlam Fashion Accessories,

Los Angeles, CA. USA

Introduction

Do you find yourself unable to have a boy child no matter how long or hard you try?

Have you been called names, or have you undergone any humiliation by those you love most or by the society because all your babies are girls?

Or maybe you have all boys and have been looking forward for a little princess?

Clueless about how to bring forth that little prince?

For those in Africa, have you wasted tons of money, going from one "prayer house"/prophet to the other in search of babies?

Do you know that there are natural methods and sex positions that give you more chances of having a baby of your choice?

What have you been eating? What has your choice of food got to do with who you conceive?

In this book I will teach you:

How to make a baby boy or a baby girl, depending on your need. You will eventually not be humiliated by others, just because all your babies are girls. Those from some parts of Africa and the East, Asia, will understand what I am talking about.

You will also learn to make a baby girl, if you have all boys.

Discover what to do to increase your man's Sperm Count.

Discover what reduces a man's Sperm Count.

Discover the different sex positions that will help you get that baby boy or girl you desire.

You will learn what foods to eat to give you more chances of conceiving a little prince.

Discover the proven scientific facts which can help you decide the gender of your baby before conception and help you ensure you get a boy or a girl.

What You Can Do To Instantly Find Out If Your Body Has The Right Environment To Conceive A Girl. This simple test you can do at home will tell you exactly how likely you are to conceive a boy or girl.

Master the several essential tips of making the baby you desire, boy or girl, which includes, the pants your man wears, if he drinks, if he smokes, the way you climax, when you climax and several more.

I wrote this book because I am burdened. I once discussed with one of my relatives that has 10 girls. 10 girls! - Since she wanted a boy. On letting her know that she can agree with her husband and make a boy, her answer was "Obu Chukwu na enye nwa!", meaning "It is God that gives a child" and she did not bother to listen to what I had to say.

I agree with her that it is God that gives children, but I also know that all it takes for us to make a baby of our choice has being given to us by God. So, it is inappropriate to fold your hands and jump on bed with your spouse to do the deed anytime you feel like, without proper and thorough planning.

You got to plan not just the sex of your baby but also the time you wish to have the baby.

I shared a lot in this book that

would help millions of women (especially in Africa and Asia-where male child is so valued) escape the humiliations of not having the baby choice they desire.

In most Asian and African countries male children are equated almost to gods.

In most families, series of abortions are committed on the news that the baby in the womb is a girl!

With this book, I intend to help stop the killings of our unborn babies.

You can plan the sex of your babies using the guidelines I will give in this book.

I am a mother of three wonderful children. Two girls and a boy.

This quest all started after the birth of my second baby girl, Vicky.

I knew from my biology class that there were ways to make a baby boy, but I never did any research on them or took them seriously.

After, I gave birth to my Vicky, I embarked on a research, as I stumbled on a newspaper that was advertising ovulation kits. I never knew that there were stuffs like that.

I got the motivation to do more research on this subject. After my findings, I planned my next pregnancy and viola! It was a boy! We named him Joshy. That was more than 8 years ago.

Since then, I have been on this journey of telling everyone I know of my new discovery.

Yes, you can create the baby you want. Yes, you can play a huge part in determining the sex of your baby.

I read that newspaper, shared my discoveries with my baby sister. Today she has three boys after the two baby girls she had initially.

I then, continued "my experiment" with my neighbors and all my friends that were in search of a baby boy. I know that some claim that these methods are not 100% accurate but, they have worked for all the women that I shared it with. My advice worked for those that heed to it.

Whenever, I had the opportunity to talk to newly engaged or newlyweds, that plan to have children, this has always been my first present - a lecture on "How to make a baby of your choice, a boy or a girl".

Much later, I started coaching women from all over the world. Many have gained success in this. They all have the babies of their choices, now.

Some of my greatest passions are to see women live a fulfilled life and for people to have marital bliss. This is also another reason I wrote this book.

I am a No.1 bestselling author of 500+ QUESTIONS YOU MUST ASK BEFORE MARRIAGE and a bestselling author of several other books which include: "FOUND BY MERCY - From the life of self-destruction to a source of inspiration", "RELATIONSHIPS 101", "LOSE 10 KG IN 10 DAYS".

I received and was nominated for several local and international awards for my works. I am also a life transformational coach, an international speaker and a TV Host.

I have helped lots of couples regain their marriages and lots of folks lose tons of weight, gaining their confidence back, through my coaching, my books on weight loss and on relationships.

Many would say, Niki, "What are you talking about?" but, I bet you to try this one, you will thank me later.

So, what are you waiting for? Get your copies and don't forget to tell others, who need this book.

Keep on reading...

Note: I am not a gynecologist or a nurse. However, I penned down my experience and results from the tons of research that I have done, that's why, in this book I will share with you actions that I took, findings, that helped me and many that I coach through the years, get the babies they desire, boy or girl.

God has given us everything to enhance our lives here on earth.

That is why we hear God say, "My people perish due to lack of knowledge".

Scroll up and click on the "buy now" button to get your copies.

The Author

Chapter 1

How to get pregnant with a boy

Are you hoping to get pregnant with a boy?

If you are desperate hoping to conceive a baby boy, there are more you can do than just crossing your fingers. As I said earlier, God has given us everything to enhance our lives here on earth. That is why we hear God say, "My people perish due to lack of knowledge". Do not be one of those that disturb God with prayers when God has already given you all that pertains to life…

There are several tips to help you get pregnant with a boy. They worked for me, my sister and worked for many that I coach through the years, as they followed all the instructions in this book.

Well, a few years ago you would just have to do your thing and hope for the best. Fortunately, today, the game has changed. Whether you want a boy or a girl, there are steps you can take to better your chances of having your desired baby. Help yourself!

From Biology Class, We Know That...

The sex of a child is determined at the moment of fertilization, when an egg containing an X chromosome encounters a sperm. That sperm can contain either a Y chromosome, in which case the embryo will be male, or an X, in which case it will be female.

If you desire a boy child, your duty however is to make the environment around an Y chromosome conducive for it to survive and get to the egg, before an X chromosome does. That environment is alkaline in nature. We will discuss this in detail in some segments below.

Firstly, let's consider the following few tips:

He Has To Wear Boxers

We both must agree together to make this happen. Boy sperms do not like heat in any way, so wearing boxers may help your man to keep things cool and breezy for the agile boys down there. Remind your man of this.

Hot tubs and hot baths Are Your Enemy For Now.
Just like tight pants and high temperature, hot baths and hot tubs can kill off the male sperms or make them less active so avoid heat.

Take Cough Syrup
If you don't want to invest in expensive medical treatments and don't want to take medicines that could have unpleasant side effects for your organism - You could try to add a few drops of cough syrup to your daily routine, as statistics show women using this trick are more likely to have baby boys. I will explain the reason given for this in the "How to Conceive a girl" section. So, read on…

A cup of coffee to the rescue!
It's a good idea for your man to drink coffee during this period

Some people swear that you can increase your chances of getting pregnant with a boy by having your man down a cup of coffee before sex. Maybe the caffeine gets those little guys swimming faster.

Consume more calories

And eat cereal for breakfast! "A study conducted by researchers at the University of Exeter in the UK suggests that upping your calorie intake by at least 400 calories per day and consuming cereal especially, along with bananas, fish, vegetables and other high energy foods, can help lead to conception of a boy," reveals Dr. Ava Cadell, spokesperson for The Experience Channel and renowned love and sex therapist. Interesting, right?

Some of the tips shared above might sound like myths but, any lady desperate for a baby boy, would try all safe ways to get him.

Without further delay, here are things I did and teach to conceive a little prince.

Know Your Ovulation Date

Do you keep records of your ovulation dates? When you plan to conceive, you want to be sure. Ovulation predictor kits are now widely available at drug and grocery stores everywhere.

I sometimes hear from couples who are trying to time their conception attempts correctly when they're trying to choose their baby's gender or sex. Many know or have read that the boy producing, or Y sperm is shorter lived than the girl producing or X sperm.

Many want clarifications as to just how long the Y sperm live and whether they can wait for the egg if you have sex before ovulation. I recently heard from a woman who said, in part: "let's say that I think that I'm going to ovulate tomorrow. If I have sex today, would the Y sperm be able to wait for my egg? Or would they die off immediately? And what does this mean if I'm trying for a boy baby?"

The answer depends upon a couple of factors, but Y or boy producing sperm are said to viable for as many as 3 days if the sperm is in the optimum alkaline environment. So, if you made it so that your vaginal tract was alkaline rather than acidic you would be prolonging the lifespan of those Y sperm to ensure that they did not die off immediately and could wait for the egg for a few days. However, if you had an acidic vaginal environment, then those same Y or boy producing sperm would likely die off much more quickly – as soon as hours later (and some Y sperm will never even make it past your vaginal tract into your fallopian tubes.)

Another consideration is how healthy and viable your partner's sperm is, and when, exactly, you have ovulated.

It's extremely common for a woman to miscalculate her ovulation day, especially if she's not using a very reliable PH tester. So, to answer the question, for the most part Y or male sperm don't die off immediately and they can wait for a short period of time for the egg. How long this period turns out to be, depends a good deal on the PH of the woman's vaginal tract.

That's why it's so very important to time your sexual intercourse correctly. This is true regardless of whether you are trying for a girl or boy baby.

It's so much better for the egg to have to wait for the sperm because the egg isn't influenced by external factors like acidity and PH.

Still confused about the easiest way to plan your conception so that you get the boy or girl baby that you want? Continue reading…

Have sex as close to ovulation as possible.

Male sperm are the faster swimmers, but they also die superfast. Female sperm can hang around for a while and take their time getting to the egg. By having sex as close to ovulation as possible, you will give male sperms a head start.

If you are in search of a baby boy, make sure to have sex on your ovulation day. Now let's find out how to be certain on this date.

When does ovulation usually occur

Ovulation usually occurs halfway through your menstrual cycle — the average cycle lasts 28 days, counting from the first day of one period (day one) to the first day of the next period. But as with everything pregnancy-related, there's a wide range of normal here (anywhere from 21 to 35 days), and your own cycle may vary slightly from month to month. For the first few years after menstruation begins, long cycles are common. However, menstrual cycles tend to shorten and become more regular as you age.

How do I know my ovulation date?

1. Check the calendar: Keep a menstrual calendar for a few months so you can get an idea of what's normal for you — or use tools that can help you calculate ovulation.

Although, personally, when we wanted to make my boy, I started charting my BBT about a week or less before my ovulation date. According to rules, your BBT jumps a bit on the start of your ovulation date and that is the right time to do the thing after considering other factors that I listed below.

If your periods are irregular, you'll need to be even more alert for other signs of ovulation, so continue reading.

2. Listen to your body: If you're like 20 percent of women, your body will send you a memo when it's ovulating, in the form of a twinge of pain or a series of cramps in your lower abdominal area (usually localized to one side — the side you're ovulating from). This is called mittelschmerz — German for "middle pain" — this monthly reminder of fertility is thought to be the result of the maturation or release of an egg from an ovary. Pay close

attention and you may be more likely to get the message. I feel mine when I pay close attention.

3. Chart your temperature: Before ovulation, your BBT (Basal Body Temperature) may range from about 36.2-36.5 degrees Celsius (97.2 to 97.7 degrees Fahrenheit). However, the day after you ovulate, you should see an uptick of 0.2 degrees F (0.11 degrees C), and then continues to rise somewhat to 1.0 degree in your BBT, which should last until your next period. (You may notice your temperature occasionally spiking on other days, but if it doesn't stay up, you probably haven't ovulated yet.) If you become pregnant, your temperature will stay elevated throughout your pregnancy.

After charting your BBT for a few months, you'll be able to see whether there's a pattern to your cycle. If there is, you may be able to estimate when you'll next ovulate. (Charting your BBT can also help your healthcare provider pinpoint the cause of fertility problems, if any arises.)

Your BBT is the baseline reading you get first thing in the morning, after at least three to five hours of sleep and before you get out of bed, talk, have sex or even sit up. Your BBT changes throughout your cycle as fluctuations in hormone levels occur. During the first half of your cycle, estrogen dominates. During the second half of your cycle (once ovulation has occurred), there is a surge in progesterone. Progesterone increases your body temperature as it gets your uterus ready for a fertilized, implantable egg. Which means that in the first half of the month, your temperature will be lower than it is in the second half of the month, after ovulation.

In other words: Your BBT will reach its lowest point at ovulation and then rise immediately and dramatically (about a half a degree) as soon as ovulation occurs. Keep in mind that charting your BBT for one month will not enable you to predict the day you ovulate but rather give you evidence of ovulation after it has occurred. Charting your BBT over a few months, however, will help you to see a pattern to your cycles, enabling you to predict when ovulation will occur in future months — and when to hop into bed accordingly. Yes, you got to catch the moment, with your man, immediately, if you are desperate for your little prince.

Talk with your man beforehand so that you will plan it together and for him to be available to jump on that bed with you.

4. Get to know your cervix: Ovulation isn't an entirely hidden process. As your body senses the hormone shifts that indicate an egg is about to be released from the ovary, it begins to ready

itself for the incoming hordes of sperm and give the egg its best chance of getting fertilized. One detectable sign of oncoming ovulation is the position of the cervix itself. During the beginning of a cycle, your cervix (that neck-like passage between your vagina and uterus that must stretch during birth to accommodate your baby's head) is low, hard, and closed. But as ovulation approaches, it pulls back up, softens a bit, and opens just a little, to let the sperm through on their way to their target. Some women can easily feel these changes, while others have a tougher time. Check your cervix daily, using one or two fingers, and keep a chart of your observations.

5. Observing the cervical mucus.

What is cervical mucus?

Cervical mucus is vaginal discharge produced by the cervix. It is that stuff that gets your underwear all sticky. Its more useful purpose is to carry the sperm to the ovum deep inside you. Over the course of your menstrual cycle, the amount, color, and texture of your cervical mucus changes, due to fluctuating hormone levels. Checking your cervical mucus and keeping track of these changes can help you tell when you're most fertile. Here's what to watch for:

Once your period stops, you may not have any discharge for a few days. Then, the mucus becomes white or cloudy appearance — and if you try to stretch it between your fingers, it'll break apart. As you get closer to ovulation, this mucus becomes even more copious, but now it's thinner, clearer, and has a slippery consistency similar to an egg white. If you try to stretch it between your fingers, you'll be able to pull it into a string a few inches long before it breaks. This consistency makes it easier for the sperm to travel through the cervix to the egg. These are your most fertile days. This is yet another sign of impending ovulation — as well as a sign that it's time to get out of the bathroom and get busy in the bedroom, when in search of a baby boy, be inseminated or to use condoms, if you are in search of a baby girl.

A good time to check your cervical mucus is when you go to the bathroom first thing in the morning, but you can check it any time of day. Sometimes you may be able to see cervical mucus on the toilet paper after you wipe. Other times you may need to insert a clean finger into your vagina (toward your cervix) to get enough mucus to examine.

Keep in mind that taking certain medications, having sex, using a lubricant, or douching can change the appearance of cervical mucus. Pay close attention to my comment on ditching in a later chapter.

To get an accurate reading, as mentioned earlier, you need to use a basal thermometer, that, which is sensitive enough to measure minute changes in body temperature. (Some experts think glass BBT thermometers are more accurate than digital ones.)

How To Measure Your BBT

My periods were regular, so I charted my BBT just for a week.

Take your temperature when you first wake up in the morning – before you eat, drink, have sex, or even sit up in bed or put a foot on the floor – and record it on a BBT chart. Try to take a reading at about the same time each morning. If you don't take your temperature immediately after waking up, your BBT chart will not be accurate. (The same is true if you get a fever.)

Ready to chart your BBT?

1. On the first day you get your period, fill in the date and day of the week under cycle day 1. Continue noting the dates of your cycle until the first day of your next period.

2. Each morning when you wake up – before you drink, eat, have sex, or even sit up in bed – take your temperature with a basal thermometer, and put a dot next to the temperature that matches your thermometer reading for that day. (You can also note the time you took your temperature. Try to take it at about the same time each morning.) Connect the dots to see how your basal temperature fluctuates from day to day.

3. You can also check your cervical mucus each day if you wish. Record the type of discharge you find each day.

4. Toward the end of your cycle, watch for a day when your BBT rose 0.5 to 1degree F and stayed high. That day is usually the day you ovulated. It should correspond with the last day you noticed egg-white type cervical mucus. The days when you notice egg-white

type mucus are your most fertile. That is the day and time to make a boy.

5. Track these symptoms for a few months to see if you notice an uptick in BBT and egg-white type mucus at the same time each cycle. That will allow you to plan which days to have sex if you want to get pregnant with a boy.

Don't like charting? Go for OPK (Ovulation Predictor Kit)

If the idea of charting sounds stressful or if you just can't make it work, there are other ways to estimate when you'll ovulate. For example, you can buy an ovulation predictor kit: Don't want to mess around with mucus? You don't have to these days. I would advise however, to do both. An ovulation predictor kit, (OPK) measures your hormone levels and indicates when you're about to ovulate. Ovulation predictor kits are able to pinpoint your date of ovulation 12 to 24 hours in advance by looking at levels of luteinizing hormone, or LH, which is the last of the hormones to hit its peak before ovulation actually occurs.

As I mentioned earlier, personally, I combined all the tips in this book and I advise you to do the same. That will get you close enough to accuracy.

How To Use An Ovulation Kit.

All you have to do is pee on a stick and wait for the indicator to tell you whether you're about to ovulate.

Silva Test

Another option is a saliva test, which takes a peek at levels of estrogen in your saliva as ovulation nears. When you're ovulating, a look at your saliva under the test's eyepiece will reveal a microscopic pattern that resembles the leaves of a fern plant or frost on a windowpane. Not all women get a good "fern," but this test, which is reusable, can be cheaper than those OPK sticks you have to pee on. There are also devices that detect the numerous salts (chloride, sodium, potassium) in a woman's sweat, which change during different times of the month, called the chloride ion surge, this shift happens even before the estrogen and the LH surge, so these tests give a woman a four-day warning of when she may be ovulating, versus the 12-to-24-hour one that the standard pee-on-a-stick OPKs provide.

The key to success in using this latest technology is to make sure to get an accurate baseline of your ion levels (currently, there's a device on the market that needs to be worn on the wrist for at least six continuous hours to get a proper baseline). Just don't forget to put together a candlelit dinner, draw a warm bubble bath, or plan a romantic weekend getaway — whatever it is that puts you and your partner in a baby-making mood.

In Summary - To Conceive a baby boy:

1. Know your ovulation date.

2. Observe your cervical mucus, if it is egg-white like, it is good time for making a boy.

3. Track your BBT, as soon it goes up a bit, (as long as you don't have fever and you measured it before sex or getting out of bed), it's time to do a boy.

4. Use OPK - Ovulation Predictor Kit, is sold everywhere and helps you know when you are ovulating.

5. Do saliva test.

I combined tips 1-4 because I did not know anything about saliva test then.

Chapter 2

Sex Positions For Making A Baby Boy. Other Sexual Attitudes That Help You Make A Boy.

The Theory:

There are two types of sperm, one carrying the X chromosome, and one carrying the Y chromosome.

The type of sperm that fertilizes the egg, and determines what sex the baby will be (X for a girl, and Y for a boy).

Dr Shettles, author of the bestselling book, How to Choose the Sex of Your Baby, believed that the types of sperm had a number of inherent differences.

Through research, he found boy sperm to be weaker, smaller and faster than their female counterparts. He discovered that female sperm were more resilient and able to survive for longer periods inside the female body.

Dr Shettles believed deep penetration was important to give the boy sperm a head start.

With less difference to travel, the boy sperm would be able to outswim the girl sperm, and find the egg.

The Shettles method claims that to improve your chances of conceiving a boy, you should have sex in positions that allow for deep penetration.

It may not sound very romantic, but the closer to the cervix the sperm are ejaculated, the more likely they are to find the egg. Here are some position which can help accomplish this:

Say Goodbye To Missionary Sex

So, it's time to say good-bye to the missionary position – at least for now, on your journey to making a baby boy. Missionary sex is for making baby girls.

You need all sex positions that will allow deeper penetration, such as:

1. Doggy Style - The position most commonly mentioned during discussions of this nature, is doggy style. This position allows for deep penetration, and is touted by many as the optimum position in which to conceive a boy. You should kneel on all fours, and have your partner enter you from behind. You could also adjust this position so that you are

kneeling or leaning over a raised surface, if you prefer.

2. Standing Up - Another position that allows for deep penetration, is sex standing up. Most standing sex positions are deep. Boy sperms are given an advantage in this position, as they swim faster against gravity to reach the egg. For this position, your partner may be able to lift you up, or you prefer to lean against a wall. Either way, you will probably need something to lean or hold onto, you don't want to end up in hospital after a sex fall.

3. The Wheelbarrow - Basically for strong women. This as the previous two, allows deep penetration.

4. Straddling

Ask your partner to lie or sit up on the bed, sofa, or wherever you choose to do the deed. You should straddle him and lower yourself onto him. This position allows for deep penetration, but with the added benefit of you being in control. If your partner has a large penis, or you feel discomfort when trying the positions above, you may prefer to be on top as this will allow you to control the depth of penetration.

"Standing sex," you on top, allow you to control the depth of penetration.

"The Wheelbarrow", which is also a form of standing sex, "Straddling" or "Doggie Style".

What is the basics of this? All these sex positions are highly recommended to couples hoping to conceive a boy. Why? "Because it allows for deeper penetration, and consequently, during ejaculation, the male sperm get deposited closer to the cervix." In general, male sperm are faster, but they don't live as long as females do, so the less distance they have to travel, the better.

Have An Orgasm!

When making a boy, a woman should not just have sex but the "big O" will make it easier for you to have a boy.

Orgasm is one of the things that helps produce a more alkaline environment that is conducive to producing boys.

Chapter 3

Vaginal Alkalinity And Your Diet

You can check how alkaline your vagina is, just by using a type of "litmus" paper called vaginal pH test strips.

For some reason, boy sperm prefer alkaline environments, which means environments that are less acidic. So, to increase alkalinity, eating more red meat, salty foods and soda are NOT recommended. Fruits, nuts, legumes and vegetables will help you achieve your goals.

Below is a list to help you.

Eat a Healthy Diet

1) Diet is usually the fix to most modern ailments, including low sperm counts. The fact is, modern diets suck. Just fixing this alone can dramatically increase your sperm count. Reducing sugars, eliminating wheat & grains and upping your fruit, vegetable & healthy fat intake is a start. This will dramatically increase your sperm count.

2) Limit Caffeine

A cup of coffee a day is not likely to reduce fertility or sperm count. But drinking caffeine in excessive amount (more than 3 cups a day) is suspected to have a negative effect on your sperm by increasing the chance of mutation.

3) Cut Back on Coke and Other Soda's

In a Danish study among 2,554 young Danish men recruited when they were examined to determine their fitness for military service, it was recorded that the men who drank high amounts of Cola had sperm counts of around 40 mL/M while the men who didn't drink Cola had an average of 56 mL/M. They couldn't say whether it was the caffeine or not, but coke and other soda are certainly not going to increase sperm counts in men, so lay off.

4) Eat Red Food

A recent study published in Ohio's Cleveland Clinic showed that consumption of Lycopene (commonly found in red fruits such as tomatoes, strawberries, cherries and peppers) increased the mobility, morphology and volume of sperm, as well as increasing sperm counts up to 70%. These findings are nothing short of amazing.

5) The Incredible Power of Garlic

Considered a natural aphrodisiac and sexual superfood, garlic contains Selenium, and antioxidant necessary for sperm motility and Allicin, and compound that increases blood flow to the male sex organs. Add it to your daily mix to see a boost in sex drive and an increase in sperm count. Just make sure you buy some chewing gum before you hit the bars. All being said, it is found that TOO MUCH garlic can actually have a negative effect on sperm counts, so use in moderation.

6) How Much Then?

For a rise in sperm count, start adding 1-2 garlic cloves to a meal daily. This will also provide you with a nice boost in libido.

7) Eat Goji Berries

A Chinese study of 42 men who were all diagnosed with infertility due to low sperm count and motility were given 15 grams or 1/2 oz of Goji Berries a day. After 1 month on the treatment 50% of the men had sperm counts in the normal and above normal range. And after only 2 months of the treatment, 33 of the men had sperm counts from normal to above normal levels and each of those 33 men went on to father children. This is amazing! Goji berries alone cando wonders for your sperm count.

Experts say as Food: Up to 30 grams of berries may be eaten daily.

8) Oyster Have Even More Sex Benefits Than We Thought

Oysters are known as being one of the most potent sexual enhancers you can naturally ingest. But what many don't know is that, as well as increasing your sex drive, they also increase your sperm count. Why is this? It is because of the extremely high amount of Zinc that oysters contain. Oysters are loaded with this building block of sperm and it will show in a rise in your swimmers.

Since Zinc is stored in our bodies there is no need to eat daily. Try eating 8-12 oysters once a week to start. Your sex that night will astound you.

9) Eat Dark Chocolate

Chocolate lovers rejoice! Dark chocolate, being loaded with antioxidants and arginine, is a potent sperm enhancer. Men who commonly eat dark chocolate also report more intense orgasms, so that's always fun. While dark chocolate does contain L-Arginine, it is not in huge amount, so learn more about how to supplement with that later.

If you like some sweets at night, start eating a few squares of dark chocolate after dinner. No need to get crazy scientific about this one.

10) Go 'Bananas'

According to Chinese traditional medicine - Functions of our body organs are enhanced by the food that look like them. So, bananas don't only look like a penis, but they make your penis better. Bananas obtain a rare enzyme called Bromelian, which is good for the bro's because it helps regulate sex hormones. They are also loaded with Magnesium, Vitamin B1 & Vitamin C, which are building blocks of sperm.

Eating 1-3 bananas a week is enough for them to help increase your sperm counts. Try it before or after a workout or sex.

11) Eat Asparagus

Asparagus contain super high levels of Vitamin C, which prevents your sperm from oxidizing, protects the cells of your testes and reduces free radical damage. They also contain Folic Acid which we will talk about later. Well worth the price of some slightly smelly urine.

Include asparagus in your dinners a few times a week. This healthy vegetable will not only improve your health, but add some class to your meals.

12) Eat More Nuts, Specifically Walnuts

Nuts have been known for a long time to be great for health as well as the male reproductive system. In 2012, a study published at the University of California showed that men who consumed 75g of walnuts every day showed a huge improvement in sperm vitality, motility and morphology (3 indicators of quality sperm). The results we concluded to be from the high amount of polyunsaturated fatty acids in nuts. Nuts like walnuts and almonds also contain a good amount of L-Arginine, which once again has been shown to increase sperm count in men while peanuts contain a good amount of Zinc. Overall, nuts are great for your nuts. Bonus: Brazilian nuts are an amazing source of Selenium that most celebrities use

to boost their testosterone and sperm count as well.

75 g of walnuts seemed to do the trick in the study. So, if you are trying to raise your sperm counts, try this amount. If you just want to get the health benefits, just start snacking on nuts regularly. For Brazilian nuts, you only need 2-3 a day to get a high dose of selenium. Don't eat more than that.

13) Try Pumpkin Seeds

Pumpkin seeds are very high in zinc, which as we spoke about above, is a major building block of sperm and testosterone. As well has containing lots of zinc, pumpkin seeds contain B vitamins, vitamin E, C, D & K which are all libido increasing vitamins. They also contain calcium, potassium, niacin and phosphorous.

Pumpkin seeds should always be eaten raw to preserve the healthy fats present. Choose organic pumpkin seeds, to avoid the harmful chemicals and pesticides which are shown to lower your sperm count & snack on them like you would sunflower seeds. Enjoy.

14) Limit Your Soy Intake

Soy and men don't collaborate. This study shows that soy dramatically reduced sperm count in men. In the study it was found that men who ate a lot of soy food had, on average, 41 million/mL less sperm than guys who didn't consume soy products. This finding is huge! And can save a lot of men from infertility problems. Stay away from soy, at all costs.

15) Eat Your Veggies

Moms are always right. Not only do cruciferous vegetables lower estrogen levels, allowing for higher testosterone levels, but they will also help you boost your sperm counts.

You should be eating veggies with EVERY meal, and be half your plate. Seriously. They will help prevent disease, increase energy, boost test & help your sperm.

16) Stay Hydrated

This is a simple solution but must be noted as the last diet point. Make sure you are staying hydrated. Your sperm is made of water and dehydration is linked to lower sperm volume. If you're doing everything else in this article, but not drinking enough water, you are doing yourself an injustice.

Drink at least 8 glasses of water daily. If you work out, then drink more.

Chapter 4

What to Avoid To Increase Sperm Count

The availability of the male sperms is directly proportional to the quality of the sperms.

High sperm count is proportional to higher chances of making a boy child.

To increase Sperm Count, help your man with the following tips:

1) Avoid Excessive Plastic Use.

BPA is used in making plastics.

BPA stands for bisphenol A. BPA is an industrial chemical that has been used to make certain plastics and resins since the 1960s. BPA is found in polycarbonate plastics and epoxy resins. Polycarbonate plastics are often used in containers that store food and beverages, such as water bottles. We use plastic excessively.

Just look around now and you will see plastics everywhere. There's no avoiding them. But as you will see everywhere, plastic chemicals like BPA and Phthalates are found in everything from our water sources to household products and are proven to decrease sperm counts.

According to research,

these chemicals came around in the 1940's, right when sperm counts began their decline. It is not a Coincidence.

Household plastics are making your man Less of a Man.

2) Don't Eat Canned Foods

According to this study, one of the plastics we referred to above, BPA, is still to this day used in many canned foods. These cans have been coated with the resin since the 1960's. BTW, BPA is known as "synthetic estrogen" and I'll be talking about it a lot in this book.

3) Say No To Receipts

Next time the clerk or ATM hands you a receipt, say "no thanks!" Once again, our little friend BPA is coated on receipts (It gives them that powdery feel). A study, where researchers got 10 people to handle unused receipts and then eat a basket of French fries, showed that, following the test, the participants had BPA levels that were 10 times higher than when they started. It's as bad as that!

4) Stop Using Most Sex Toys

Sex toys are often made with the plastic softening chemicals called phthalates. These phthalates are proven to lower sperm count. How can you stay safe while still having fun? Stick to glass, silicone and green sex toys. If in fact, you need them at all. Talk to your spouse to give you a "sex treat" I don't like sex toys. I believe it's not a necessity or maybe I am too "old school" or religious)

5) Use Natural Lube

Most lubricants are not sperm friendly. They either kill the sperm or they can act like a barrier and are too thick for the sperm to swim through. This is bad for couples trying to conceive and can make your sperm much less effective. Luckily there are sperm friendly lubricants created for just that. So, search for those.

6) Watch Out For Non-Stick Pans & Raincoats

Weird combination, but these two things contain chemicals called perfluoroalkyl acids which give them their non-stick quality. It was found that men with high levels of these chemicals in their blood (like plant workers) had half the sperm counts of normal men.

7) Shower Naturally

Phthalates are found in most shampoos, soaps, conditioners, deodorants and shaving products. They make you feel silky smooth, but they are destroying your sperm count. You can increase your sperm count simply by switching to organic products that are phthalate free. It will be worth the extra 20 penny a month when you can father children and make the baby of your choice.

8) Avoid Other Harmful Chemicals

I have said enough about chemicals. For the sake of everyone, we'll end it here. So basically, just watch out for chemicals in general. Pesticides and other harmful chemicals all play a role in sperm count reduction. These chemicals wreak havoc on our endocrine systems, and put our swimmers at risk. You can find these on most fruits and veggies that are not certified organic. For best results, just buy organic. Also, all those crazy cleaning products you use. Stick to organic products as much as possible. Just this alone will increase your sperm count. Use vinegar, lemon and baking soda instead, for cleaning.

9) Stop Smoking Dope

Studies show that marijuana smokers have significantly less seminal fluid and a decreased sperm count. Some herbs are deadly. Marijuana smoking damages sperm.

10) Stop Smoking

If you want to increase your sperm count you have to ditch the cigarettes. This should be the first thing you do.

11) Check Your Medications

Many common medications can lower your sperm count. When trying to boost sperm counts, make sure you Google search "any medications you are taking + sperm count." This will quickly tell you if these medications are some of the many that interfere with sperm counts.

13) Get That Laptop Off Your Lap!

A hot laptop on your lap is a recipe for sperm loss. Excessive heat + Testicles = Bad for baby making business. Use a pillow or buy a lap desk and ensure your 'boys' are nice and cool, like you.

14) Attention - Wifi!

Another reason to get that laptop off your lap is because a recent study showed that blasting sperm collected from 29 healthy men with wifi exposure caused one-quarter of the sperm to stop swimming, while only 14% of sperm not exposed stopped swimming. This is alarming.

15) Stay Sober

While alcohol is not shown to drastically decrease sperm counts, it is a good strategy to limit the booze when you are trying to increase your sperm count or father children.

16) Bike Less

It was found in a study of Spanish triathletes that they had a lower sperm count than athletes competing in sports that didn't involve cycling. The study showed that there was an inverse relationship between the shape of the head, tail and body of the spermatozoids and hours spent cycling each week.

17) Watch Less T.V

A recent study showed that men who watched 20 hours of T.V or more a week had half the sperm of men who didn't watch T.V at all. This is a startling statistic. If you want to increase your sperm count, turn off the tube.

18) Move Your Cellphones Off Your Pockets

The fact is, cell phones emit radiation in the form of electromagnetic waves. Having this go on in your pocket, which is RIGHT next to your balls, is a horrible combination.

You can increase your sperm count simply by keeping your phone in an armband rather than your pocket.

19) Watch Out For Hot Baths & Hot Tubs

Hot tubs are awesome. But they are not good for your sperm whatsoever. Just 30 minutes in water that is 38,8 C (102 F) or higher will significantly lower your immediate sperm count. Studies done in the 1950's show that men who took a half hour hot bath every other day for 3 weeks were infertile for the next six months!

On top of that, a recent study done at UCSF(The University of California, San

Francisco) showed that when men cut out their exposure to hot baths, their sperm counts went up 491%. That is huge!

20) Exercise

Exercise seems to be good for everything, and this is no different when it comes to increasing your sperm count. A study shows that men exercising more than 7 hours a week had roughly 48% higher concentrations in sperm than men who exercised less than 1 hour per week.

21) Lose Weight

The good news is, if you're exercising, you probably have this one covered. Studies show that being obese (having a BMI over 30) greatly decreases a man's chance of being fertile while also lowering his sperm count.

Male Infertility is More Common in Overweight Men.

22) Have More Sex

What good news! Recent researches show that using your sperm doesn't make it any less potent. And it's the opposite. "Saving your sperm" for when a woman is more fertile is a bad strategy. According to research, guys with low sperm counts who abstain for more than a day slow down production even more and cause the sperm that is in the bank to go "stale." Enjoy your sex. Have Sex Daily to Boost Sperm Count.

23) Practice Deep Breathing

Deep breathing supplies the body with much more oxygen than shallow breathing. This makes cells come alive and the sperm cells are not exceptions.

24) Loosen The Super Tight Undies

In order for the testes to produce quality sperm, the temperature of the testes must be much lower than your body temperature. This is why your balls are located outside of your body. Even a couple degrees in temperature rise is enough to have a negative effect, so if they are tight enough to be holding your balls too close to your body (this means super tight), they will hurt your sperm count, even if only slightly.

25) Take Cold Showers

Cold showers are great for you. They increase your insulin resistance, have been shown to ease depression, boost testosterone levels, help you sleep better at night, and yes, increase sperm counts. I know it sounds terrible, but try it. It really does wake you up in the morning like nothing else. Ironically it also helps you to sleep at night like nothing else. Just do it.

Chapter 5

Supplements That Increase Sperm Count.

1)Take Folic Acid

A study on Folic Acid and Zinc's effect on fertile and sub fertile men resulted in a 74%

increase in sperm counts in the sub fertile men who supplemented both for two weeks. A simple solution for any man lacking sperm.

2) Take Zinc

As mentioned above, Zinc was part of that study were sub fertile men boosted their sperm counts by 74%. Zinc is one of the major players in increasing sperm count and deficiency is becoming more and more widespread every year.

3) Take L-Carnitine

According to Italian Researchers, Carnitine helps sluggish sperm. In a study they did, men took 2 grams of L-Carnitine daily for three months and then took none for 3 more months. The men who took the L-Carnitine over the placebo experienced an improvement in sperm motility, a crucial factor in fertility.

Sperm Swim Better With L-Carnitine

4) Take Selenium

As mentioned in the "eat more nuts" section, you can get a full dose of selenium just by consuming Brazilian Nuts. But if for some reason you hate eating nuts, it would be very wise to supplement with Selenium. This will boost your testosterone, increase your sperm count and possibly prevent Cancer. Take

2-3 Brazil Nuts daily.

5) Take Vitamin E

Vitamin E is another critical antioxidant in the production of sperm. In this study, along with Selenium it was proven to improve the quality of your sperm.

In the above study, the men took 400 mg of vitamin E daily.

6) Take L-Arginine

L-Arginine is the amino acid found in nuts which is one of the reasons they are regarded as huge sperm boosters. L-Arginine will increase your sperm count and motility, and has been proven to do so in numerous studies. Along with this, it will increase blood flow to your penis resulting in better erection quality. Overall L-Arginine is a fantastic addition to any mans supplement regimen.

How Much?

According to research, start with 1000mg daily. You can increase this amount safely up to 5,000 mg but some find this to be too much.

7) Take Tongkat Ali Extract

Tongkat ali extract is man most potent sexual enhancer. This herb is proven to increase libido, boost testosterone, increase sperm count, increase sperm volume, increase ejaculation power, decrease your refractory period & much more. A study of 75 men who cycled tongkat ali extract for 9 months showed a dramatic improvement in all semen parameters.

8) Take Maca

Maca is another potent male enhancing herb that you may not be taking advantage of. In 2001, the Asian Journal of Andrology released a study showing that Maca increased the seminal volume, sperm motility and sperm count in men. A year later, they released a 12-week study on males between the age of 20 and 55 which showed that after 12 weeks all men not in the placebo group noted an improvement in libido.

9) Take Ginseng

Ginseng is an extremely popular sperm enhancer. It is also shown to improve blood flow to the penis and help improve erection quality, energy levels and much more.

When opting for Ginseng, choose Asian Ginseng (also known as Korean Ginseng or Panax Ginseng). Asian ginseng should also be taken in cycles. For example, take every day for 2 – 3 weeks, then stop for 3 weeks, then start back. Take 200mg to 400mg daily.

10) Don't Take Public Enemy #1 for Male Fertility: Anabolic Steroids

As listed under medications that lower Sperm Count - Steroids are harmful… And to top off the list, if you think that taking steroids will make you more of a man, you are wrong. While it will increase the size of your muscles, taking steroids is proven to reduce the amount and quality of your sperm.

11) Massaging the point in the picture helps to increase Sperm Count.

In Conclusion

Remember, it takes 10-11 weeks for sperm to be produced. So, you cannot just try some of the things listed above and expect to have super sperm by tomorrow morning. These things take time. But even knocking 40% of these things off your list will be enough to give you a dramatic increase in your sperm count. Want the best sperm in the world? Then try all that I mentioned to eat, avoid all that I listed to avoid and remind your man of the supplements too.

Chapter 6

16 Common Medications That Can Lower Your Sperm Count You Should Avoid.

Speak to your doctor if you are on any of these medications and want to find a safe alternative:

1) Anabolic Steroids / Testosterone Therapy can actually make men permanently sterile, cutting sperm count and quality.

2) Antidepressants like Prozac, Paxil, and Zoloft can alter libido and the ability to get an erection or ejaculate. These drugs may also damage sperm and make them unable to fertilize an egg.

3) Antifungal medications can lower sperm count.

4) Ketoconazole can inhibit the production of hormones.

5) Blood pressure medications. Antihypertensive potassium-sparing diuretics can impact male fertility by diminishing the sperm's ability to fertilize an egg.

6) Calcium channel blockers, such as Plendil, Cardene, Procardia, Cardiol, Cardizem, and Verapamil, can lower sperm count.

7) Chemotherapy drugs can lower sperm count. Talk to your doctor about any alkylating agents you may be taking, including cyclophosphamide, nitrogen mustard, and methotrexate.

8) Diuretics can cause dehydration and lead to low semen volume.

9) Epilepsy drugs like Carbamazepine and Valproate can lower sperm count and decrease testosterone.

10) Heart medications, ask your doctor

Painkillers can inhibit prostaglandin release and delay ovulation, decrease libido and cause ejaculatory dysfunction.

11) Propecia. This can affect male reproductive hormones enough to weaken sperm production and function, especially in men with sperm counts that are low or borderline to begin with.

12) Sulfasalazine, used to treat IBS, Ulcerative Colitis, Crohn's disease, can also reduce sperm count.

13) Tranquilizers can impact sperm count

Ulcer medications for peptic ulcers: Cimetidine can lower sperm count in men and cause increased prolactin which impairs male fertility.

14) Urinary function drugs Nitrofurantoin (Macrodantin) can lower sperm count.

15) Viagra. At Queen's University in Belfast Ireland researchers found that a single 100 milligram dose of Viagra can prematurely activate the acrosome on the head of the sperm. It's the little sack of enzymes that makes the outer membrane of the egg dissolve a little so that the sperm can penetrate the egg. If the acrosome pops off too soon, it won't do its duty at the right time.

16) Herbal Viagra. Avoid internet herbs that claim to be "herbal Viagra" as they treat the symptoms, not the root cause and won't help.

Chapter 7

Summary Of How to Conceive A Boy

A male sperm will most likely fertilize the egg if you:

1. Have intercourse 12 hours before ovulation. The male sperms can swim faster and reach the egg before the female sperm

2. Track your ovulation signs using an ovulation kits and know when you are about to ovulate.

- Chart your BBT
- Observe your cervical mucus – egg white like mucus is for swaying boys.

3. Have intercourse using a sexual position (e.g. Doggy style) that causes deep penetration.

4. Follow a specific diet that causes the cervical mucus pH to be more alkaline.

5. Remind your man to avoid hot baths and tubs.

Remember..

To conceive a boy, you need to eat foods that help your body become more alkaline:

1. Do not eat dairy products because they make your cervical mucus sticky and unfriendly to sperm.

2. Eat freshly squeezed juices once or twice a day (avoid store bought juices that are pasteurized, make your own at home using a juicer).

3. Eat lots of fresh vegetables (make sure they are lightly steamed or raw, otherwise they will lose their minerals and vitamins)

4. Eat foods that are high in potassium (bananas, avocados, prunes, dried apricots, and figs)

5. Eat foods that make your body more alkaline.

Earlier, I gave a list of supplements that increases the Sperm Count in men. However, Evening Primrose Oil, a Supplements for ladies will double your chances of conceiving A Boy

"Evening Primrose Oil increases the quality of cervical mucus and help support male sperm survival in the female reproductive tract."

Male sperm is weaker than female sperm and survives for a shorter period of time once released. It needs to get to the egg first and as soon as possible. On a good note, male sperm can swim faster than female sperm. So, if the woman's fertile mucus is high in quantity, male sperm can be nourished to survive longer.

Evening Primrose Oil increases fertile mucus production and it should be taken when your menses stop until ovulation.

If you know you do not produce enough fertile cervical mucus, you need to take a supplement like FertileCM to increase production of healthy fertile mucus. While conceiving a boy, it is important to have lots of cervical mucus to support male sperm survival.

Ovulation And Timing: Do Not Miss This!

To increase your chances of having a male sperm reach the egg, time intercourse right at ovulation. If you do not know exactly when you ovulate, you need to learn how to chart your fertility signs in order to detect ovulation. I've explained how to chart both BBT and other things. Go back and read that.

Ovulation kits can definitely help you achieve this task. A fertility monitor can help you detect your fertile days 5-7 days in advance.

Remember: timing is the key!

Once you know you are about to ovulate, have intercourse at least 12-24 hours before ovulation. The closer to ovulation you have intercourse, the higher your chances of conceiving a baby boy.

Why? Because the male sperm swim faster than the female sperm. Also, male sperm does not live as long, so you need to have sex often and as close as possible to ovulation. If you manage to have intercourse just before ovulation, lots of healthy male sperm will be ready to fertilize the egg once it is released from the ovary.

If you have intercourse right on the day before your ovulation, the male sperm will reach the egg first because they swim faster and because there will be lots of them. The likelihood of conceiving a boy greatly increases to almost 100%.

Female Orgasm When Conceiving A Boy

The women should reach orgasm during intercourse when trying to conceive a boy. Having an orgasm changes the pH level of the cervical mucus to a more alkaline value. An alkaline environment increases the survival rate of the male sperm.

Also, a low pH or acidic pH will cause the male sperm to die sooner than the female one, which can survive longer in an acidic environment.

The Father's Role

I took time to explain what the men can eat, avoid and supplements they can take to ensure that he increases his Sperm Count.

Now that you know that you have a quality sperm and that your sperm count is high, it is also important to ejaculate as many times as possible, right before/on ovulation day.

The idea here is to release sperm in the female reproductive tract only at ovulation to have as many male sperm as possible. By ejaculating for a number of times on the ovulation day or hours before, the sperm count increases and the likelihood of having male sperm is higher. This is contrary to what experts taught decades ago.

The father should also avoid warming up the testicles because male sperm less resistant to heat than female sperm. The father should avoid having a sauna or using a hot tub while trying to conceive a boy, warm showers are fine.

Bicycling should also avoid as this can cause overheating of the genital area. Many doctors also advise against tight-fitting underwear for the same reason.

"If the male partner has low sperm count, it is important to help increase by avoiding drugs, alcohol, illness, stress, coffee, toxic exposure, smoking, and cell phones. Increase moderate levels of regular exercise."

Vaginal pH When Conceiving a Boy: Get It Right!

The pH of the vagina should be alkaline in order to support male sperm. In fact, male sperms need an environment that is NOT acidic. In order to check the pH of your cervical mucus, you can purchase at your local health food store pH strips and test just before ovulation.

If your pH is acidic you need to increase it to alkaline levels through your diet by eating alkaline forming foods.

Douching

Douching with baking soda is recommended only in women who are extremely acidic. Add two tablespoons of baking soda in lukewarm water, mix gently and allow the enough time for the baking soda to be completed dissolved.

Apply the douche using a disposable douche bottle from the pharmacy. Make sure to rinse thoroughly to avoid contamination. Many practitioners do not recommend extensive douching while trying to conceive.

Though personally, I am against douching of any sort. I remember how I suffered yeast infection for a long time due to this. The doctors prescribed all kinds of douching and drugs. However, my predicament did not stop until I stopped douching and changed my diet. The vagina cleanses itself. Do not interfere with that. Avoid douching, unless of course, only at this time you are in the boy swaying process. I believe that it is best to make your vagina alkaline by eating the right kind of food first, as stated above.

My Advice

If you really want to conceive a baby boy, don't forget to read the whole book. By the time you finish reading this entire book without missing any detail, you will find out sure-fire strategies that will help you to conceive a baby boy.

Imagine the fun you'll have when going shopping for new baby boy clothes!

I truly hope you succeed and have a healthy baby boy!

I know how most couples in Africa and Asia, due to tradition, really want to have a baby boy. I once knew a woman who had 9 girls and each time she wanted a boy. She desperately wanted to give her husband the boy he desired. I wish I knew then what I know now about conceiving a boy, I would have been able to give her some advice.

Chapter 8

Methods For Having a Sweet Baby Girl

The Secret To Gender Selection.

As I explained in the above chapters, the sperm responsible for conceiving a girl carry the X chromosome. They are much larger, more durable and though they may take longer to reach an egg, they have a greater chance of living long enough to do so. They prosper in an acidic environment.

How To Select The Right Time To Have Sex And Make Sure You Conceive A Girl.

It is very important to know when is the absolute best time for you to get pregnant with a baby girl.

You should engage in sexual intercourse about three to four days prior to the start of your ovulation as this will be the best time if you are trying to have a girl. The reasoning behind this is that the sperms which carry X chromosomes or the ones responsible for a girl baby, are much stronger than the sperms which carry Y chromosomes or the responsible for a boy baby. The male chromosomes would die by the time when the egg would be ready to collect the sperm, and this will increase the chances of getting pregnant with a girl. You should avoid having sex on the day of ovulation or the day after.

The O +12 method (Ovulation plus 12 day)

Here it is considered that if you have a regular cycle, doing the deed 12 days after your ovulation will give you a baby girl.

Easy Sex Positions Which Highly Boost The Chances Of Having A Baby Girl.

It's been said that the missionary position is best when engaging in intercourse to have a baby girl as it is one of the ways to increase the chances. This position allows shallow penetration, so the woman's vagina entrance will be less alkaline. The X chromosomes can survive in a highly acidic environment, but it will be difficult for Y chromosomes. As such, this will increase your chances of getting pregnant with a baby girl.

Have a hot bath, both of you!
As we learnt earlier cold bath is good for boy sperms and so having a hot bath prior to sex may help to weaken the male sperm awaiting release. So, if you want a girl, soak yourself and your man in a hot tub before the deed.

Eating for a baby Girl

Low salt diet

Salt is thought to be bad for female sperm.

In order to have a girl, you need to focus on foods that will boost acidity in your body.

They include foods that are rich in magnesium and calcium. Broccoli is the perfect example of a food that contains high levels of both. Other foods you can eat include grapefruit, apples, dairy products, some fish (farm raised to avoid high levels of mercury) and leafy green vegetables.

These foods may alter the consistency, composition and pH of your vagina, making it friendlier to female sperm and increasing their lifespan.

Sex Positions That You Must Keep Away From, To Make a Baby Girl.

The doggy style, the wheelbarrow, struggling and other sex positions that allow deep penetration should be avoided. These positions increase the chances of getting pregnant with a baby boy. So, you must strictly avoid them if you want a girl baby. Missionary sex position is one of the good positions for a girl, since it doesn't allow deep penetration.

Missionary position is having sex lying down in the man-on-top position. It gives shallow penetration. Supposedly male sperm don't survive well in acidic environments. As a woman's vagina is more acidic nearer the entrance, deep penetration helps male sperm avoid the area.

Just Say "No" to the Big O

Sorry ladies, if you want a baby girl you have to say no to the big O for now.

It seems unfair, but there are two explanations for this. When a woman climaxes, she releases a substance that increases alkaline levels in her vagina. As male sperm prefer alkaline environments, it gives them more chance of survival. And orgasms help move sperm towards the cervix, so faster swimming male sperm have more chance of reaching the egg.

Many moms claim pregnant sex is the best they've had due to increased blood flow down below.

Cough Medicine Is Bad For Making Baby Girls.

It is assumed that, the guaifenesin in your cough syrup that thins your nasal mucus works in your girly parts too. As you already read from the how to Conceive a boy part of the book, that is supposedly more favorable for Y-chromosome (boy) sperm. So, if you plan to make a baby girl this cough syrup is No, No!

Woman Be In Charge On Bed During Baby Making Period

As a woman you know when the signs are conducive. You charted your BBT and cervical mucus so you should suggest sex when the time and conditions are perfect.

This also works for making baby boys.

However, for the best chance of conceiving ANY BABY SEX (BOY or GIRL) is to have sex at least, every other day during your most fertile period.

Congratulations for reading the whole book,

You have done all you know how to do, now you are qualified for miracles!

Blessings….

www.ingramcontent.com/pod-product-compliance
Lightning Source LLC
Chambersburg PA
CBHW070302230526
45470CB00002B/688